55 Juice Recipes to Control Your Eating After You Quit Smoking:

Get through the Tough Times Using Natural Solutions

By

Joe Correa CSN

COPYRIGHT

This publication is designed to provide accurate and authoritative information in regard to the subject matter covered. It is sold with the understanding that neither the author nor the publisher is engaged in rendering medical advice. If medical advice or assistance is needed, consult with a doctor. This book is considered a guide and should not be used in any way detrimental to your health. Consult with a physician before starting this nutritional plan to make sure it's right for you.

ACKNOWLEDGEMENTS

This book is dedicated to my friends and family that have had mild or serious illnesses so that you may find a solution and make the necessary changes in your life.

55 Juice Recipes to Control Your Eating After You Quit Smoking:

Get through the Tough Times Using Natural Solutions

By

Joe Correa CSN

CONTENTS

ABOUT THE AUTHOR

After years of Research, I honestly believe in the positive effects that proper nutrition can have over the body and mind. My knowledge and experience has helped me live healthier throughout the years and which I have shared with family and friends. The more you know about eating and drinking healthier, the sooner you will want to change your life and eating habits.

Nutrition is a key part in the process of being healthy and living longer so get started today. The first step is the most important and the most significant.

INTRODUCTION

55 Juice Recipes to Control Your Eating After You Quit Smoking: Get through the Tough Times Using Natural Solutions

By Joe Correa CSN

It's no secret that smoking is one of the leading causes of death in the world. This habit has some devastating effects on the entire body, your immune system, respiratory tract, and even your cardiovascular system. Not to mention the effects cigarettes have on your skin, teeth, and nails. Unfortunately, we are all aware of these facts but somehow we still decide to start smoking hoping that it won't happen to us.

Lighting a cigarette might seem like a perfect conversational starter or a good addition to your morning coffee. However, it's a well-known fact that over 400,000 people die from lung cancer and cardiovascular diseases in the United States alone. These poor statistics should be and probably are the main reason you have decided to quit smoking.

Getting rid of cigarettes is the best decision for your overall health and well-being. Unfortunately, it's not an easy decision and changes don't happen overnight. In this difficult period of life, you will have to work hard to improve your health and go through all the side-effects of your decision such as food cravings, mood swings, and similar. These are quite normal and you should be well-prepared to deal with them in the best possible manner.

In this difficult period, you will experience low blood sugar and other metabolic changes that might add some additional stress to your recovery process. This is when food becomes very important in your life as it helps you control your cravings, gives you the opportunity to enjoy something besides cigarettes, and finally, keeps you happy and satisfied.

The best way to help your body get back on track after you have quit smoking, is to plan your nutrition carefully. Wise food choices, carefully planned meal plans and some extra nutrients through juicing will help reduce your cravings and ease the detoxification process.

This book is a fantastic collection of juice recipes that will help you control your eating after you have stopped smoking. The recipes in this book are based on powerful natural ingredients that have the ability to detoxify your body and clean your entire organism. These healthy and delicious juices will give you the necessary strength you need in order to stay away from cigarettes once and for all. Take a few minutes every morning to prepare one of these spectacular juices. Get started now!

55 JUICE RECIPES TO CONTROL YOUR EATING AFTER YOU QUIT SMOKING: GET THROUGH THE TOUGH TIMES USING NATURAL SOLUTIONS

1. Apple Celery Juice

Ingredients:

1 large Granny Smith's apple, cored and chopped

2 large celery stalks, chopped

1 medium-sized peach, pitted and chopped

2 whole plums, pitted and chopped

Preparation:

Wash the apple and cut in half. Remove the core and cut into bite-sized pieces. Set aside.

Wash the celery stalks and chop into small pieces. Set aside.

Wash the peach and cut in half. Remove the pit and chop into small pieces. Set aside.

Wash the plums and remove the pits. Chop into bite-sized pieces and set aside.

Now, combine apple, celery, peach, and plums in a juicer. Process until well juiced. Transfer to a serving glass and add some ice.

Serve immediately.

Nutrition information per serving: Kcal: 209, Protein: 4.1g, Carbs: 61.3g, Fats: 1.4g

2.   Zucchini Squash Juice

Ingredients:

1 medium-sized zucchini, peeled and chopped

1 cup of butternut squash, cubed

1 cup of cucumber, thinly sliced

1 cup of avocado, peeled and chopped

1/4 tsp of cinnamon, ground

Preparation:

Peel the zucchini and chop into small pieces. Set aside.

Cut the butternut squash in half. Scoop out the seeds and then peel one half. Cut into small cubes and fill the measuring cup. Reserve the rest in the refrigerator.

Wash the cucumber and cut into thin slices. Set aside.

Peel the avocado and cut in half. Remove the pit and chop into small pieces. Fill the measuring cup and reserve the rest in the refrigerator.

Now, combine zucchini, butternut squash, cucumber, and avocado in a juicer. Process until juiced and transfer to a serving glass. Stir in the cinnamon and refrigerate for 10 minutes before serving.

Enjoy!

Nutrition information per serving: Kcal: 390, Protein: 8.7g, Carbs: 43.9g, Fats: 34.5g

3. Cauliflower Broccoli Juice

Ingredients:

1 cup of cauliflower, chopped

2 cups of broccoli, chopped

1 cup of asparagus, trimmed and chopped

2 oz of coconut water

Preparation:

Trim off the outer leaves of the cauliflower. Chop into small pieces and fill the measuring cup. Reserve the rest for later.

Wash the broccoli and trim off the outer leaves. Chop into small pieces and fill the measuring cup. Reserve the rest in the refrigerator.

Wash the asparagus and trim off the woody ends. Chop into small pieces and fill the measuring cup. Set aside.

Now, combine cauliflower, broccoli, and asparagus in a juicer. Process until well juiced. Transfer to a serving glass and stir in the coconut water.

Refrigerate for 10-15 minutes before serving.

Enjoy!

Nutrition information per serving: Kcal: 390, Protein: 8.7g, Carbs: 43.9g, Fats: 34.5g

4.   Cranberry Pineapple Juice

Ingredients:

1 cup of cranberries

1 cup of pineapple, chopped

1 medium-sized apple, chopped

1 cup of apricot, sliced

Preparation:

Using a large colander, rinse the cranberries under cold running water. Drain and fill the measuring cup. Reserve the rest for later.

Using a sharp cutting knife, cut the top and peel the pineapple. Chop into small cubes and fill the measuring cup. Reserve the rest in the refrigerator for some other juice.

Wash the apple and cut in half. Remove the core and cut into bite-sized pieces. Set aside.

Wash the apricot and cut in half. Remove the pit and chop into small pieces. Set aside.

Now, combine cranberries, pineapple, apple, and apricot in a juicer. Process until well juiced. Transfer to a serving glass and add some ice cubes.

Serve immediately.

Nutrition information per serving: Kcal: 248, Protein: 4.3g, Carbs: 76.1g, Fats: 1.3g

5. Cinnamon Banana Juice

Ingredients:

1 large banana, peeled and chunked

1 medium-sized Red Delicious apple, cored

1 whole plum, cored

¼ tsp of cinnamon, ground

2 oz of coconut water

Preparation:

Peel the banana and cut into small chunks. Set aside. Wash the apple and cut lengthwise in half. Remove the core and cut into bite-sized pieces. Set aside.

Wash the plum and cut in half. Remove the pit and cut into bite-sized pieces. Set aside.

Now, combine banana, apple, and plum in a juicer and process until well juiced. Transfer to a serving glass and stir in the coconut water and cinnamon.

Add few ice cubes before serving and enjoy!

Nutrition information per serving: Kcal: 238, Protein: 2.5g, Carbs: 68.4g, Fats: 1.1g

6.   Cucumber Honey Juice

Ingredients:

1 medium-sized cucumber, sliced

1 tbsp honey, raw

1 cup of strawberries, chopped

1 cup of spinach, torn

2 oz of water

Preparation:

Wash the cucumber and cut into thin slices.

Wash the strawberries and remove the stems. Cut into bite-sized pieces and set aside.

Wash the spinach thoroughly under cold running water. Slightly drain and torn into small pieces. Set aside.

Now, combine cucumber, strawberries, and spinach in a juicer and process until juiced. Transfer to a serving glass and stir in the water and honey.

Garnish with some mint, but it's optional.

Refrigerate for 10 minutes before serving.

Enjoy!

Nutrition information per serving: Kcal: 83, Protein: 6.9g, Carbs: 24.6g, Fats: 1.3g

7.   Apricot Cucumber Juice

Ingredients:

1 cup of apricots

1 large cucumber, sliced

1 cup of pineapple, chunked

1 cup of fresh spinach, torn

1 whole lemon

½ cup of raw broccoli, chopped

½ cup of pure coconut water

Preparation:

Wash the apricots and cut in half. Remove the pit and chop into chunks. Set aside.

Wash the cucumber and chop into thick slices. Set aside.

Cut the top of a pineapple and peel it using a sharp knife. Cut into small chunks and reserve the rest in the refrigerator.

Peel the lemon and cut lengthwise in half. Set aside.

Combine spinach and broccoli in a colander and wash

under cold running water. Drain and roughly chop. Set aside.

Now, process apricots, cucumber, pineapple, lemon, spinach, and broccoli in a juicer. Transfer to serving glasses and stir in the coconut water.

Add some ice and serve immediately.

Nutrition information per serving: Kcal: 218, Protein: 10g, Carbs: 64g, Fats: 1.9g

8.   Asparagus Collard Greens Juice

Ingredients:

1 cup of fresh asparagus, chopped

1 cup of collard greens, torn

1 large peach, chopped

1 large grapefruit, peeled

1 cup of Romaine lettuce, shredded

1 cup of fennel, sliced

Preparation:

Wash the asparagus and trim off the woody ends. Chop into small pieces and set aside.

Combine collard greens and lettuce in a colander and wash under cold running water. Torn with hands and set aside.

Wash the peach and cut in half. Remove the pit and cut into bite-sized pieces. Set aside.

Peel the grapefruit and cut into small pieces. Set aside.

Wash the fennel bulb and trim off the wilted outer layers. Cut into small chunks and set aside.

Now, combine asparagus, collard greens, peach, lettuce, grapefruit, and fennel in a juicer and process until juiced.

Transfer to serving glasses and add some ice before serving.

Nutrition information per serving: Kcal: 187, Protein: 9.1g, Carbs: 57.9g, Fats: 1.4g

9.   Blackberry Turnip Juice

Ingredients:

1 cup of fresh blackberries

1 cup of turnip greens, chopped

1 cup of plums, halved

½ tsp of ginger, ginger

1 tsp of coconut sugar

½ cup of water

Preparation:

Wash the blackberries under cold running water. Set aside.

Wash the turnip greens and torn with hands. Set aside.

Wash the plums and cut in half. Remove the pits and set aside.

Now, combine blackberries, turnip greens, and plums in a juicer. Process until juiced.

Transfer to a serving glass and stir in the coconut sugar, ginger, and water.

Refrigerate for 10 minutes before serving.

Enjoy!

Nutrition information per serving: Kcal: 141, Protein: 4.2g, Carbs: 40.3g, Fats: 1.4g

10.   Orange Radish Juice

Ingredients:

1 large orange, peeled

1 cup of radishes, chopped

1 medium-sized apple, peeled and wedged

1 cup of Iceberg lettuce, torn

1 cup of watercress, chopped

1 tbsp of honey, raw

Preparation:

Peel the orange and divide into wedges. Set aside.

Wash the radishes and trim off the green parts. Cut into small pieces and fill the measuring cup. Set aside.

Wash the apple and cut in half. Remove the core and chop into small pieces. Set aside.

Rinse the lettuce and watercress. Drain and torn with hands.

Now, combine orange, radishes, apple, lettuce, and watercress in a juicer and process until juiced.

Transfer to serving glasses and add some ice before serving.

Enjoy!

Nutrition information per serving: Kcal: 150, Protein: 7.3g, Carbs: 53.4g, Fats: 0.8g

11.   Cranberry Honey Juice

Ingredients:

1 cup of fresh cranberries

1 tbsp of honey, raw

2 cups of cherries, pitted

1 cup of leek, chopped

1 tbsp of fresh mint, finely chopped

Preparation:

Rinse the cranberries and cherries under cold running water using a colander. Drain and set aside.

Cut the cheries into halves. Remove the pits and set aside.

Wash the leek and cut into small pieces. Set aside.

Combine cranberries, cherries, leek, and mint in a juicer and process until juiced.

Transfer to serving glasses and stir in the honey.

Add some ice and serve!

Nutrition information per serving: Kcal: 248, Protein: 5g, Carbs: 75.5g, Fats: 1g

12. Coco Apricot Juice

Ingredients:

1 cup of apricots, sliced

½ cup of pure coconut water, unsweetened

1 tbsp of coconut sugar

1 cup of mango, chopped

Preparation:

Wash the apricots and cut in half. Remove the pits and chop into small pieces. Set aside.

Peel the mango and cut into small chunks. Fill the measuring cup and rserve the rest in the refrigerator.

Now, combine apricots, mango, and coconut water in a juicer. Process until juiced.

Transfer to serving glasses and stir in the coconut sugar.

Add few ice cubes and serve immediately.

Nutrition information per serving: Kcal: 155, Protein: 3.6g, Carbs: 43g, Fats: 1.2g

13. Cauliflower Fennel Juice

Ingredients:

1 cup of cauliflower, chopped

1 cup of fennel, sliced

1 cup of beet greens, chopped

1 cup of celery, chopped

1 cup of red leaf lettuce, shredded

1 cup of romaine lettuce, shredded

1 large grapefruit

½ cup of pure coconut water

1 tsp of honey

Preparation:

Trim off the outer leaves of cauliflower. Wash it and cut into small pieces. Reserve the rest in the refrigerator.

Wash the fennel bulb and trim off the wilted outer layers. Cut into small chunks and set aside.

Combine beet greens, red leaf lettuce, and Romaine lettuce in a colander and wash under cold running water.

Drain and chop roughly with hands. Set aside.

Peel the grapefruit and divide into wedges. Set aside.

Wash the celery and cut into small pieces. set aside.

Now, process cauliflower, fennel, beet greens, celery, lettuce, and grapefruit in a juicer. Transfer to serving glasses and stir in the coconut water and honey.

Add some ice and serve!

Nutrition information per serving: Kcal: 163, Protein: 8.3g, Carbs: 56.3g, Fats: 1.2g

14.   Spinach Peach Juice

Ingredients:

1 large peach, chopped

1 cup of baby spinach, torn

2 large Golden delicious apples, peeled and seeds removed

½ cup of water

1 large carrot, sliced

½ whole lemon

Preparation:

Wash the peach and cut in half. Remove the pit and chop into small pieces. Set aside.

Wash the baby spinach thoroughly and torn with hands. Set aside.

Wash the apples and cut in half. Remove the core and cut into bite-sized pieces. Set aside.

Wash the carrot and cut into thick slices. Set aside.

Peel the lemon and cut lengthwise in half. Reserve the rest for later.

Now, combine peach, spinach, apples, peach, carrot, and lemon in a juicer and process until juiced.

Transfer to serving glasses and refrigerate for 10 minutes before serving.

Nutrition information per serving: Kcal: 297, Protein: 5.5g, Carbs: 87.5g, Fats: 1.5g

15.   Banana Spinach Juice

Ingredients:

1 large banana, peeled

1 cup of spinach, torn

2 whole lemons, peeled

1 slice of ginger root, peeled

1 tsp of honey

Preparation:

Peel the banana and chop into chunks. Set aside.

Rinse the spinach thoroughly under cold running water using a colander. Drain and torn with hands. Set aside.

Peel the lemons and cut lengthwise in half. Set aside.

Peel the ginger root and finely chop it. Set aside.

Combine banana, spinach, lemons, and ginger in a juicer and process until juiced.

Transfer to serving glasses and stir in the honey.

Add some ice and serve.

Nutrition information per serving: Kcal: 139, Protein: 4.5g, Carbs: 44.4g, Fats: 1.2g

16.   Kiwi Apple Juice

Ingredients:

2 large kiwis, peeled

1 medium-sized apple, cored

1 cup of fresh spinach

1 large cucumber

1 small ginger root slice, 1-inch

Preparation:

Peel the kiwis and cut lengthwise in half. Set aside.

Wash the apple and remove the core. Cut into bite-sized pieces and set aside.

Wash the spinach thoroughly and torn with hands. Set aside.

Wash the cucumber and cut into thick slices. Set aside.

Peel the ginger root slice and set aside.

Now, process spinach, kiwis, apple, cucumber and ginger in a juicer.

Transfer to a serving glass and add some ice before

serving.

Nutrition information per serving: Kcal: 201, Protein: 13.2g, Carbs: 56.5g, Fats: 2.6g

17. Strawberry Orange Juice

Ingredients:

1 cup of fresh strawberries

1 large orange, peeled

1 cup of fresh cranberries

2 oz of coconut water

Preparation:

Combine strawberries and cranberries in a colander and wash under cold running water. Drain and set aside.

Peel the orange and divide into wedges. Set aside.

Combine cranberries, strawberries, and orange in a juicer and process until juiced.

Transfer to serving glasses and stir in the coconut water.

Add some ice and serve immediately.

Nutrition information per serving: Kcal: 137, Protein: 3.1g, Carbs: 46.7g, Fats: 0.7g

18.   Watermelon Honey Juice

Ingredients:

1 cup of watermelon, seeded

1 tbsp of liquid honey

1 cup of fresh blueberries

1 cup of fresh raspberries

1 cup of fresh cranberries

1 large lemon, peeled

Preparation:

Cut the watermelon lengthwise. For one cup, you will need about 1 large wedge. Peel and cut into chunks. Remove the seeds and set aside. Reserve the rest of the melon for some other juices.

Combine blueberries, raspberries, and cranberries in a colander and wash under cold running water. Drain and set aside.

Peel the lemon and cut lengthwise in half. Set aside.

Now, process watermelon, blueberries, raspberries, cranberries, and lemon in a juicer. Transfer to serving glasses and stir in the liquid honey.

Add some ice cubes before serving.

Enjoy!

Nutrition information per serving: Kcal: 230, Protein: 4.1g, Carbs: 53.1g, Fats: 1.7g

19.   Ginger Squash Juice

Ingredients:

1 tsp of ginger, ground

1 cup of acorn squash, cubed

1 cup of pumpkin, cubed

1 cup of butternut squash, cubed

1 large cucumber

Preparation:

Wash the crookneck squash and cut in half. Scoop out the seeds using a spoon. Cut into small chunks and set aside. Reserve the rest for another juice.

Peel the pumpkin and cut in half. Scoop out the seeds using a spoon. Cut one large wedge and peel it. Cut into small chunks and set aside. Reserve the rest for later.

Peel the butternut squash and remove the seeds using a spoon. Cut into small cubes and reserve the rest of the squash for some other recipe. Wrap in a plastic foil and refrigerate.

Wash the cucumber and cut into thick slices. Set aside.

Now, combine crookneck squash, pumpkin, butternut squash, and cucumber in a juicer and process until juiced. Transfer to serving glasses and stir in the ginger.

Add some ice and serve immediately.

Nutrition information per serving: Kcal: 140, Protein: 5.8g, Carbs: 40.1g, Fats: 0.9g

20. Kale Watercress Juice

Ingredients:

1 fennel bulb, trimmed

1 cup of fresh kale

1 cup of watercress

1 cup of fresh basil

1 large cucumber

3 tbsp of fresh parsley

A handful of spinach

Preparation:

Combine kale, watercress, basil, parsley, and spinach in a colander and wash under cold running water. Drain and torn with hands. Set aside.

Wash the fennel bulb and trim off the wilted outer layers. Cut into small chunks and set aside.

Wash the cucumber and cut into thick slices. Set aside.

Now, process kale, watercress, fennel, basil, parsley, spinach, and cucumber in a juicer.

Transfer to serving glasses and stir in the Cayenne pepper. You can add some salt but this is optional.

Refrigerate for 10 minutes before serving.

Nutrition information per serving: Kcal: 280, Protein: 6.1g, Carbs: 84.2g, Fats: 1.3g

21. Tomato Beet Juice

Ingredients:

1 medium-sized Roma tomato, chopped

1 cup of beets, trimmed

1 cup of fresh basil, torn

1 tsp of ginger, ground

1 tbsp of fresh parsley, chopped

Preparation:

Wash the tomato and place in a bowl. Cut into quarters and reserve the juice while cutting. Set aside.

Wash the beets and trim off the green parts. Cut into small pieces and set aside.

Wash the basil thoroughly and torn with hands. Set aside.

Now, process tomato, beets, basil, and ginger in a juicer.

Transfer to a serving glass and refrigerate for 10 minutes before serving.

Enjoy!

Nutrition information per serving: Kcal: 99, Protein: 6.4g, Carbs: 28.7g, Fats: 1.2g

22.   Cherry Apple Juice

Ingredients:

1 cup of fresh cherries, pitted

2 large red apples, cored

1 large banana, chopped

1 cup of watercress

A handful of fresh spinach

Preparation:

Wash the cherries under cold running water. Drain and cut in half. Remove the pits and set aside.

Wash the apple and cut in half. Remove the core and chop into small pieces. Set aside.

Peel the banana and cut into small chunks. Set aside.

Combine watercress and spinach in a colander and wash thoroughly. Torn with hands and set aside.

Now, combine cherries, apples, banana, watercress, and spinach in a juicer and process until juiced.

Transfer to serving glasses and add few ice cubes before serving.

Enjoy!

Nutrition information per serving: Kcal: 390, Protein: 6.6g, Carbs: 113g, Fats: 1.7g

23.   Zucchini Watermelon Juice

Ingredients:

1 medium-sized zucchini, peeled and chopped

1 cup of watermelon, diced

2 cups of green grapes

1 slice of ginger, 1-inch

1 tbsp of fresh mint, finely chopped

Preparation:

Wash the zucchini and cut in half. Scoop out the seeds using a spoon. Cut into small chunks and set aside.

Cut the watermelon lengthwise. For one cup, you will need about one large wedge. Peel and cut into chunks. Remove the seeds and set aside. Reserve the rest of the melon for some other juices.

Wash the grapes under cold running water. Drain and set aside.

Peel the ginger slice and set aside.

Now, process zucchini, watermelon, grapes, and ginger in a juicer.

Transfer to serving glasses and garnish with mint.

Refrigerate for 10 minutes before serving.

Nutrition information per serving: Kcal: 308, Protein: 5.7g, Carbs: 81.3g, Fats: 2.1g

24.   Apple Yam Juice

Ingredients:

2 medium-sized green apples, cored

1 small sweet potato, peeled

2 large carrots, sliced

1 large orange, peeled

¼ tsp of pumpkin pie spice

Preparation:

Wash the apples and cut in half. Remove the core and chop into bite-sized pieces. Set aside.

Peel the potato and place in a pot of boiling water. Cook for 5 minutes, or until soften. Remove from the heat and drain. Set aside to cool.

Wash the carrot and cut into thin slices. Set aside.

Peel the orange and divide into wedges. Cut each wedge in half and set aside.

Now, combine apples, potato, carrot, and orange in a juicer. Process until juiced. Transfer to serving glasses and stir in the pumpkin spice.

Add some ice cubes and serve immediately.

Enjoy!

Nutrition information per serving: Kcal: 147, Protein: 2.1g, Carbs: 35.4g, Fats: 0.1g

25.   Apple Chia Juice

Ingredients:

2 large apples, cored

1 tbsp of chia seeds

3 large carrots, sliced

½ tsp of ginger, ground

Preparation:

Wash the apples. Cut in half and remove the core. Cut into bite-sized pieces and set aside.

Wash and cut the carrots into thin slices. Set aside.

Now, process in a juicer until well juiced. Transfer to serving glasses and stir in the chia seeds.

Refrigerate for 10 minutes to allow chia to soak up the liquid. Add a little bit of water to adjust the thickness, if needed.

Enjoy!

Nutrition information per serving: Kcal: 177, Protein: 3.2g, Carbs: 28.4g, Fats: 4.6g

26. Squash Broccoli Juice

Ingredients:

½ yellow squash, peeled and chopped

1 medium-sized broccoli, chopped

½ cup of fresh kale

1 large apple, cored

¼ cup of fresh spinach

4 small carrots

Preparation:

Peel the squash and cut in half. Scoop out the seeds and chop into bite-sized pieces. Reserve the remaining half in the refrigerator.

Wash and chop the broccoli and carrots. Combine it with squash.

Wash and core the apple. Chop into bite-sized pieces and add to the remaining prepared ingredients.

Combine spinach and kale in a medium bowl and add water enough to cover it. Soak for 15 minutes.

Now, combine squash, broccoli, apple, and carrots in a

juicer. Drain the kale and spinach and add it to the juicer. Process until well juiced.

Transfer to serving glasses and refrigerate for 10 minutes before serving.

Enjoy!

Nutrition information per serving: Kcal: 81, Protein: 2.3g, Carbs: 18.4g, Fats: 0.2g

27.   Cucumber Celery Juice

Ingredients:

1 large cucumber, sliced

1 celery stalk, chopped

½ cup of fresh kale

1 large lime, peeled

Preparation:

Wash and chop the cucumber and celery. Add it to the bowl with lime.

Soak the kale in water for 15 minutes. Set aside.

Peel the lime and cut into bite-sized pieces. Place it in a bowl and set aside.

Drain the kale and process it with cucumber, lime, and celery.

Transfer to serving glasses and refrigerate for a while, or add some ice and serve immediately.

Nutrition information per serving: Kcal: 171, Protein: 3.2g, Carbs: 47.3g, Fats: 1.3g

28.   Pear Lime Juice

Ingredients:

1 large pear, cored

1 lime, peeled

1 cup of green grapes

2 large cucumbers, sliced

Preparation:

Wash the pear and remove the core. Cut into bite-sized pieces and set aside.

Peel the lime and cut into quarters. Set aside.

Wash the green grapes under cold running water and drain using colander. Set aside.

Wash the cucumbers and cut into thin slices. Set aside.

Now, combine pear, lime, grapes and cucumber in a juicer. Process until juiced. Transfer to serving glasses and stir well.

Refrigerate for 10 minutes before serving.

Enjoy!

Nutrition information per serving: Kcal: 113, Protein: 18.3g, Carbs: 31.3g, Fats: 0.1g

29.   Carrot Lemon Juice

Ingredients:

3 large carrots, sliced

1 large lemon, peeled

1 medium-sized cucumber, sliced

1 large pear, cored

¼ cup of fresh mint

½ cup of broccoli, chopped

1 small ginger root slice, 1-inch

½ tsp of green tea powder

2 oz of water

Preparation:

Wash the carrots and cut into small pieces. Set aside.

Peel the lemon and cut into quarters. Set aside.

Wash and cut the cucumber into small pieces. Set aside.

Wash the pear and remove the core. Cut into bite-sized pieces and set aside.

Combine broccoli and mint in a colander and wash under cold running water. Drain and set aside.

Peel the ginger root and set aside.

Combine tea powder and hot water in a small cup. Let it stand for 5 minutes.

Now, combine carrots, lemon, cucumber, pear, mint, broccoli, and ginger root slice in a juicer. Process until nicely juiced.

Transfer to serving glasses and stir in the tea mixture.

Refrigerate for 5 minutes before serving.

Nutrition information per serving: Kcal: 141, Protein: 5.5g, Carbs: 45.7g, Fats: 0.9g

30.   Strawberry Carrot Juice

Ingredients:

1 cup of fresh strawberries, chopped

1 large carrot, sliced

1 medium-sized green apple, cored and chopped

1 medium orange, wedged

1 cup of cucumber, sliced

Preparation:

Wash the strawberries and remove the top stems. Cut into small pieces and set aside.

Wash the carrot and cut into thin slices. Set aside.

Wash the apple and cut in half. Remove the core and cut into bite-sized pieces. Set aside.

Peel the orange and divide into wedges. Set aside.

Wash the cucumber and cut into thin slices. Set aside.

Now, process strawberries, carrots, apple, orange, and cucumber in a juicer. Transfer to the serving glasses refrigerate for 5 minutes before serving.

Enjoy!

Nutrition information per serving: Kcal: 104, Protein: 3.9g, Carbs: 31.2g, Fats: 1.1g

31. Cucumber Apple Juice

Ingredients:

1 large cucumber, sliced

1 large red apple, cored

2 medium-sized beets, trimmed

1 large lime, peeled

¼ tsp of ginger, ground

Preparation:

Wash the cucumber and cut it into thick slices. Set aside.

Wash the apple and remove the core. Cut into bite-sized pieces and set aside.

Wash the beets and trim off the green ends. Save it for another juice. Cut the beet into small pieces. Set aside.

Peel the lime and cut into quarters. Set aside.

Now, process cucumber, apple, beets, and lime in a juicer. Transfer to serving glasses and add some ice before serving.

Enjoy!

Nutrition information per serving: Kcal: 109, Protein: 2.8g, Carbs: 33.6g, Fats: 0.7g

32.   Apple Lemon Juice

Ingredients:

1 green apple, cored

1 large lemon, peeled

1 large broccoli, chopped

1 large cucumber, sliced

¼ tsp of peppermint extract

½ cup of fresh mint

Preparation:

Wash the apple and remove the core. Cut into bite-sized pieces and set aside.

Peel the lemon and cut into quarters. Set aside.

Wash the broccoli and cut into small pieces. Set aside.

Wash the cucumber and cut into thick slices. Set aside.

Wash the fresh mint and soak in water for 5 minutes.

Now, combine apple, lemon, broccoli, cucumber, and mint in a juicer and process until juiced.

Transfer to serving glasses and stir in the peppermint

extract.

Garnish with some extra mint leaves and add some ice before serving.

Enjoy!

Nutrition information per serving: Kcal: 191, Protein: 2.3g, Carbs: 28.4g, Fats: 1.7g

33.   Apricot Pomegranate Juice

Ingredients:

2 large apricots, pitted

1 cup of pomegranate seeds

2 large oranges, peeled

1 cup of green grapes

1 large lemon, peeled

1 small ginger slice, peeled

Preparation:

Wash the apricots and cut in half. Remove the pits and cut into small pieces. Set aside.

Cut the top of the pomegranate fruit using a sharp knife. Slice down to each of the white membranes inside of the fruit. Pop the seeds into a measuring cup and set aside.

Peel the oranges and divide into wedges. Set aside.

Peel the lemon and cut lengthwise in half. Set aside.

Peel the ginger slice and set aside.

Now, combine apricots, pomegranate, oranges, lemon,

and ginger in a juicer. Process until well juiced and transfer to serving glasses. Refrigerate for 20 minutes before serving.

Nutrition information per serving: Kcal: 294, Protein: 7.2g, Carbs: 88.9g, Fats: 2.3g

34.   Apple Cucumber Juice

Ingredients:

1 large red apple, cored

1 large cucumber, sliced

1 cup of blueberries

1 cup of fresh mint, torn

2 oz of coconut water

Preparation:

Wash the apple and cut in half. Remove the core and cut into bite-sized pieces. Set aside.

Wash the cucumber and gently peel it. Cut into thin slices and set aside.

Place the blueberries in a colander and wash under cold running water. Drain and set aside.

Wash the mint thoroughly and torn with hands. Set aside.

Now, combine apple, cucumber, blueberries, and mint in a juicer. Process until juiced and transfer to serving glasses. Stir in the coconut water and refrigerate for 10 minutes, or add some ice before serving.

Enjoy!

Nutrition information per serving: Kcal: 258, Protein: 4.7g, Carbs: 74.6g, Fats: 1.6g

35.   Raspberry Kiwi Juice

Ingredients:

1 cup of raspberries

1 large kiwi, peeled

2 cups of watermelon, chopped

1 large orange, peeled

2 oz coconut water

Preparation:

Wash the raspberries thoroughly under cold running water. Drain and set aside.

Peel the kiwi and cut lengthwise in half. Set aside.

Cut the watermelon lengthwise. For two cups, you will need about two large wedges. Peel and cut into chunks. Remove the seeds and set aside. Reserve the rest of the melon for some other juices. Set aside.

Peel the orange and divide into wedges. Set aside.

Now, combine raspberries, kiwi, watermelon, and orange in a juicer. Process until juiced and transfer to serving glasses. Stir in the coconut water and refrigerate for 10 minutes before serving.

Nutrition information per serving: Kcal: 232, Protein: 5.8g, Carbs: 71.4g, Fats: 1.8g

36.   Parsnip Parsley Juice

Ingredients:

1 cup of parsnip, sliced

1 tbsp of fresh parsley, chopped

3 large red bell peppers, chopped

1 cup of butternut squash, cubed

2 oz of water

Preparation:

Wash the parsnip and peel it. Cut into thin slices and set aside.

Wash the red bell peppers and cut lengthwise in half. Remove the seeds and chop into small pieces.

Peel the butternut squash and remove the seeds using a spoon. Cut into small cubes and fill the measuring cup. Reserve the rest of the squash for some other recipe. Wrap in a plastic foil and refrigerate.

Now, combine parsnip, parsley, bell peppers, and butternut squash in a juicer. Process until well juiced and transfer to serving glasses. Stir in the water and add some ice.

Serve immediately.

Nutrition information per serving: Kcal: 238, Protein: 7.9g, Carbs: 70.2g, Fats: 2.1g

37.   Pomegranate Apple Juice

Ingredients:

1 cup of pomegranate seeds

1 large green apple, cored and chopped

1 large papaya, peeled and chopped

1 tbsp of fresh mint, chopped

2 oz of water

Preparation:

Cut the top of the pomegranate fruit using a sharp knife. Slice down to each of the white membranes inside of the fruit. Pop the seeds into a measuring cup and set aside.

Wash the apple and cut in half. Using a sharp knife, remove the core and cut into bite-sized pieces. Set aside.

Peel the papaya and cut lengthwise in half. Scoop out the black seeds and flesh using a spoon. Cut into small chunks and set aside.

Now, combine pomegranate, apple, papaya, and mint in a juicer. Process until well juiced and transfer to serving glasses. Stir in the water and refrigerate for 10 minutes before serving.

Enjoy!

Nutrition information per serving: Kcal: 438, Protein: 6.1g, Carbs: 129g, Fats: 3.4g

38.   Lime Guava Juice

Ingredients:

1 cup of pineapple chunks

2 large limes, peeled

1 cup of guava, chopped

1 large cucumber, sliced

1 tbsp of fresh basil, chopped

2 oz of water

Preparation:

Peel the limes and cut lengthwise in half. Set aside.

Wash the guava and cut into chunks. Fill the measuring cup and reserve the rest for some other recipe in a refrigerator.

Cut the top of a pineapple and peel it using a sharp knife. Cut into small chunks and fill the measuring cup. Reserve the rest of the pineapple in a refrigerator.

Wash the cucumber and cut into thin slices. Set aside.

Now, combine limes, guava, pineapple, cucumber, and basil in a juicer. Process until well juiced and transfer to serving glasses. Stir in the water and refrigerate for 10 minutes before serving.

Nutrition information per serving: Kcal: 158, Protein: 4.7g, Carbs: 47.9g, Fats: 1.1g

39.   Apple Nutmeg Juice

Ingredients:

1 large green apple, cored

¼ tsp of nutmeg, ground

1 cup of cranberries

1 large pear, cored

3 large strawberries, chopped

1 large orange, peeled

2 oz of coconut water

Preparation:

Wash the apple and cut in half. Remove the core and cut into bite-sized pieces. Set aside.

Wash the cranberries thoroughly under cold running water. Drain and set aside.

Wash the pear and cut lengthwise in half. Remove the core and cut into bite-sized pieces. Set aside.

Wash the strawberries thoroughly and chop into small pieces. Set aside.

Peel the orange and divide into wedges. Set aside.

Now, combine pear, apple, strawberries, orange, and nutmeg in a juicer. Process until well juiced and transfer to serving glasses.

Stir in the water and refrigerate or add some ice before serving.

Nutrition information per serving: Kcal: 158, Protein: 4.7g, Carbs: 47.9g, Fats: 1.1g

40.   Collard Greens Watercress Juice

Ingredients:

1 cup of collard greens, torn

1 cup of watercress, torn

1 cup of asparagus, trimmed

1 green bell pepper, chopped

1 large cucumber, sliced

2 oz of water

¼ tsp of salt

Preparation:

Combine collard greens and watercress in a colander. Wash thoroughly under cold running water and torn with hands. Set aside.

Wash the asparagus and trim off the woody ends. Cut into bite-sized pieces and fill the measuring cup. Reserve the rest for some other juice.

Wash the bell pepper and lengthwise in half. Remove the seeds and chop into small pieces. Set aside.

Wash the cucumber and cut into thin slices. Set aside.

Now, combine collard greens, watercress, asparagus, bell pepper, and cucumber in a juicer and process until well juiced. Transfer to serving glasses and stir in the salt and water.

Refrigerate for 10 minutes before serving.

Nutrition information per serving: Kcal: 86, Protein: 8.2g, Carbs: 26.1g, Fats: 1g

41. Swiss Chard Lettuce Juice

Ingredients:

1 cup of Swiss chard, torn

1 cup of red leaf lettuce, torn

1 cup of sweet potatoes, peeled

1 large fennel, chopped

1 cup of fresh spinach, torn

1 small cauliflower head, chopped

1 large lemon, peeled

Preparation:

Combine Swiss chard, red leaf lettuce, and spinach in a colander. Wash under cold running water and drain. Torn with hands and set aside.

Peel the sweet potato and cut into small chunks. Fill the measuring cup and reserve the rest for some other juice.

Wash the fennel bulb and trim off the wilted outer layers. Cut into small chunks and set aside.

Trim off the outer leaves of cauliflower. Wash it and cut into small pieces. Set aside.

Peel the lemon and cut lengthwise in half. Set aside.

Now, combine Swiss chard, lettuce, potato, fennel, cauliflower, and lemon in a juicer and process until well juiced. Transfer to serving glasses and add some ice before serving.

Nutrition information per serving: Kcal: 218, Protein: 14.3g, Carbs: 67.7g, Fats: 1.9g

42.   Pepper Cucumber Juice

Ingredients:

1 large yellow bell pepper, chopped

1 large cucumber, sliced

1 medium-sized fennel bulb, chopped

1 cup of Brussels sprouts, halved

¼ tsp of salt

2 oz of water

Preparation:

Wash the bell pepper and cut lengthwise in half. Remove the seeds and chop into small pieces. Set aside.

Wash the cucumber and cut into thin slices. Set aside.

Trimm off the fennel stalks and wilted outer layers. Cut into bite-sized pieces and set aside.

Trim off the outer leaves and wash the Brussels sprouts. Cut in half and set aside.

Now, combine bell peppers, cucumber, fennel, and Brussels sprouts in a juicer. Process until well juiced and stir in the salt and water. Refrigerate for 5 minutes before serving.

Nutrition information per serving: Kcal: 151, Protein: 9.7g, Carbs: 47.6g, Fats: 1.4g

43.   Blackberry Cucumber Juice

Ingredients:

1 cup of blackberries

1 large cucumber, sliced

5 whole plums, pitted

1 cup of purple cabbage, chopped

2 oz of water

Preparation:

Wash the blackberries under cold running water using a colander. Slightly drain and set aside.

Wash the cucumber and cut into thin slices. Set aside.

Wash the plums and cut in half. Remove the pits and cut into quarters. Set aside.

Wash the cabbage thoroughly under cold running water. Drain and roughly chop it. Set aside.

Now, combine plums, cabbage, blackberries, and cucumber in a juicer and process until juice. Transfer to serving glasses and stir in the water.

Refrigerate for 10 minutes before serving.

Nutrition information per serving: Kcal: 221, Protein: 7.5g, Carbs: 69.1g, Fats: 2.1g

44.   Beet Basil Juice

Ingredients:

1 cup of beets, chopped

1 cup of fresh basil, torn

2 cups of raspberries

1 large green apple, cored

1 large lemon, peeled

3 oz of water

Preparation:

Wash the beets and trim off the green ends. Cut into small pieces and fill the measuring cup. Reserve the greens for some other juice.

Wash the basil thoroughly under cold running water and torn with hands. Set aside.

Wash the raspberries under cold running water using a colander. Drain and set aside.

Wash the apple and cut in half. Remove the core and cut into bite-sized pieces. Set aside.

Peel the lemon and cut lengthwise in half. Set aside.

Now, combine beets, basil, raspberries, apple, and lemon in a juicer. Process until well juiced.

Stir in the water and refrigerate for 5 minutes before serving.

Enjoy!

Nutrition information per serving: Kcal: 218, Protein: 7.5g, Carbs: 76.4g, Fats: 2.5g

45.   Pomegranate Lemon Juice

Ingredients:

1 cup of pomegranate seeds

1 large lemon, peeled

1 large apricot, pitted

1 large orange, wedged

1 large carrot, peeled

2 oz of coconut water

Preparation:

Cut the top of the pomegranate fruit using a sharp knife. Slice down to each of the white membranes inside of the fruit. Pop the seeds into measuring cup and set aside.

Peel the lemon and cut lengthwise in half. Set aside.

Wash the apricot and cut in half. Remove the pit and cut into small pieces. Set aside.

Peel the orange and divide into wedges. Set aside.

Peel and wash the carrot. Cut into thin slices and set aside.

Now, combine pomegranate seeds, lemon, apricot, orange, and carrot in a juicer. Process until well juiced and transfer to serving glasses. Stir in the coconut water and add few ice cubes before serving.

Nutrition information per serving: Kcal: 241, Protein: 7.3g, Carbs: 73.9g, Fats: 2.3g

46.   Kale Parsley Juice

Ingredients:

1 cup of fresh kale, torn

1 cup of fresh parsley, torn

2 cups of broccoli, trimmed

1 large green apple, chopped

1 cup of fresh spinach, torn

2 oz of water

Preparation:

Combine kale, parsley, and spinach in a colander and wash under cold running water. Drain and torn with hands. Set aside.

Wash the broccoli under cold running water and cut into small pieces. Set aside.

Wash the apple and cut in half. Remove the core and cut into bite-sized pieces. Set aside.

Now, combine kale, parsley, broccoli, apple, and spinach in a juicer. Process until well juiced and stir in the water.

Refrigerate for 10 minutes before serving.

Nutrition information per serving: Kcal: 223, Protein: 20.4g, Carbs: 62.1g, Fats: 3.5g

47.   Apple Strawberry Juice

Ingredients:

1 large red apple, cored

2 large strawberries, chopped

2 large grapefruits, peeled

1 small ginger knob, peeled

2 oz of coconut water

Preparation:

Wash the apple and cut in half. Remove the core and cut into bite-sized pieces. Set aside.

Wash the strawberries and cut into small pieces. Set aside.

Peel the grapefruits and divide into wedges. Set aside.

Peel the ginger knob and set aside.

Now, combine apple, strawberries, grapegfruit, and ginger in a juicer. Process until well juiced and transfer to serving glasses. Stir in the coconut water and refrigerate for 10 minutes before serving.

Enjoy!

Nutrition information per serving: Kcal: 302, Protein: 4.8g, Carbs: 86.3g, Fats: 1.7g

48. Cucumber Swiss Chard Juice

Ingredients:

1 large cucumber, sliced

1 cup of Swiss chard, torn

2 cups of pumpkin, cubed

1 large green apple, cored

2 oz of water

¼ tsp of nutmeg, ground

Preparation:

Wash the cucumber and cut into thin slices. Set aside.

Wash the Swiss chard thoroughly under cold running water. Drain and torn with hands. Set aside.

Peel the pumpkin and cut in half. Scoop out the seeds using a spoon. Cut one large wedge and peel it. Cut into small cubes and fill the measuring cup. Reserve the rest for some other juice.

Wash the apple and cut in half. Remove the core and cut into bite-sized pieces. Set aside.

Now, combine pumpkin, apple, cucumber, and Swiss

chards in a juicer. Process until well juiced and stir in the water and nutmeg.

Refrigerate for 10 minutes before serving.

Nutrition information per serving: Kcal: 196, Protein: 5.8g, Carbs: 55.4g, Fats: 1.1g

49.   Bean Mint Juice

Ingredients:

1 cup of green beans, chopped

1 cup of fresh mint, torn

2 cups of celery, chopped

1 cup of beet greens, torn

1 large cucumber, sliced

2 oz of water

¼ tsp of salt

Preparation:

Wash the green beans and cut into bite-sized pieces. Soak in hot water for 10 minutes. Drain and set aside.

Wash the celery and cut into small pieces. Set aside.

Combine mint and beet greens in a colander. Wash under cold running water and torn with hands. Set aside.

Wash the cucumber and cut into thin slices. Set aside.

Now, combine green beans, mint, celery, beet greens, and cucumber in a juicer. Process until well juiced and transfer to a serving glass. Stir in the water and salt.

Refrigerate for 5 minutes before serving.

Nutritional information per serving: Kcal: 91, Protein: 6.1g, Carbs: 26.1g, Fats: 1g

50.   Lemon Kiwi Juice

Ingredients:

1 large lemon, peeled

1 large kiwi, peeled

1 cup of strawberries, chopped

2 large peaches, pitted

1 large green apple, cored

1 large orange, peeled

2 oz of water

Preparation:

Peel the lemon and kiwi. Cut lengthwise in half and set aside.

Wash the strawberries under cold running water. Remove the green parts and cut into bite-sized pieces. Set aside.

Wash the peaches and cut in half. Remove the pits and cut into small pieces. Set aside.

Wash the apple and cut half. Remove the core and cut into bite-sized pieces. Set aside.

Now, combine, lemon, kiwi, strawberries, peaches, and apple in a juicer and process until well juiced. Transfer to serving glasses and stir in the water. Add some ice and serve immediately.

Enjoy!

Nutrition information per serving: Kcal: 345, Protein: 7.8g, Carbs: 105g, Fats: 2.3g

51.   Raspberry Apricot Juice

Ingredients:

1 cup of raspberries

3 large apricots, pitted

1 cup of blackberries

1 large red apple, cored

3 large carrots, peeled

Preparation:

Combine raspberries and blackberries in a colander. Wash under cold running water and slightly drain. Set aside.

Wash the apricots and cut in half. Remove the pits and cut into bite-sized pieces. Set aside.

Wash the apple and cut in half. Remove the core and cut into small pieces.

Wash and peel the carrots. Cut into thin slices and set aside.

Now, combine blackberries, raspberries, apricots, apple, and carrots in a juicer. Process until well juiced and transfer to serving glasses. Stir in the water and

refrigerate for 10 minutes before serving.

Enjoy!

Nutrition information per serving: Kcal: 301, Protein: 7.6g, Carbs: 97.4g, Fats: 2.9g

52.   Avocado Mint Juice

Ingredients:

1 cup of avocado, pitted

1 cup of fresh mint, chopped

1 cup of strawberries, chopped

1 large Granny Smith's apple, cored and chopped

1 large lemon, peeled

1 large cucumber, sliced

Preparation:

Peel the avocado and cut lengthwise in half. Remove the pit and cut into chunks and fill the measuring cup. Reserve the rest for later.

Wash the mint thoroughly and torn with hands. Set aside.

Wash the strawberries and cut into small pieces. Set aside.

Wash the apple and cut in half. Remove the core and cut into bite-sized pieces. Set aside.

Peel the lemon and cut lengthwise in half. Set aside.

Wash the cucumber and cut into thin slices. Set aside.

Now, combine avocado, mint, strawberries, lemon, and cucumber in a juicer and process until juiced. Transfer to serving glasses and stir in the water. Add some ice and serve immediately.

Nutrition information per serving: Kcal: 376, Protein: 8.1g, Carbs: 67.8g, Fats: 23.3g

53.　　Cranberry Plum Juice

Ingredients:

1 cup of cranberries

4 whole plums, pitted

1 cup of pomegranate seeds

1 large red bell pepper, chopped

1 large green apple, cored

Preparation:

Wash the cranberries thoroughly and drain. Set aside.

Wash the plums and cut in half. Remove the pits and cut into bite-sized pieces. Set aside.

Cut the top of the pomegranate fruit using a sharp knife. Slice down to each of the white membranes inside of the fruit. Pop the seeds into a measuring cup and set aside.

Wash the bell pepper and cut lengthwise in half. Remove the seeds and cut into small pieces. Set aside.

Wash the apple and cut in half. Remove the core and cut into bite-sized pieces. Set aside.

Now, combine cranberries, plums, pomegranate, and

apple in a juicer. Process until well juiced and add some ice before serving.

Enjoy!

Nutrition information per serving: Kcal: 277, Protein: 6g, Carbs: 83g, Fats: 1.4g

54.   Blueberry Cucumber Juice

Ingredients:

1 cup of blueberries

1 large cucumber, sliced

1 cup of mango, chopped

1 large green apple, cored

2 oz of water

Preparation:

Place the blueberries in a colander and wash under cold running water. Drain and set aside.

Wash the cucumber and cut into thin slices. Set aside.

Wash the mango and cut into chunks. Fill the measuring cup and reserve the rest for some other juice. Set aside.

Wash the apple and remove the core. Cut into bite-sized pieces and set aside.

Now, combine blueberries, cucumber, mango, and apple in a juicer and process until juiced.

Transfer to serving glasses and stir in the water. Add some ice before serving and enjoy!

Nutrition information per serving: Kcal: 180, Protein: 5.9g, Carbs: 63.5g, Fats: 1.1g

55.   Celery Mint Juice

Ingredients:

1 cup of celery, chopped

1 cup of fresh mint, chopped

1 large lemon, peeled

1 cup of fresh spinach, chopped

2 oz of water

Preparation:

Wash the celery stalks and chop into small pieces. Fill the measuring cup and set aside.

Peel the lemon and cut lengthwise in half. Set aside.

Wash the spinach and mint in a colander. Chop and place in a medium bowl. Set aside.

Now, combine celery, lemon, mint, and spinach in a juicer and process until juiced.Transfer to serving glasses and stir in the water.

Refrigerate for 5 minutes before serving.

Nutrition information per serving: Kcal: 35, Protein: 3.1g, Carbs: 13.2g, Fats: 0.7g

ADDITIONAL TITLES FROM THIS AUTHOR

70 Effective Meal Recipes to Prevent and Solve Being Overweight: Burn Fat Fast by Using Proper Dieting and Smart Nutrition

By Joe Correa CSN

48 Acne Solving Meal Recipes: The Fast and Natural Path to Fixing Your Acne Problems in Less Than 10 Days!

By Joe Correa CSN

41 Alzheimer's Preventing Meal Recipes: Reduce or Eliminate Your Alzheimer's Condition in 30 Days or Less!

By Joe Correa CSN

70 Effective Breast Cancer Meal Recipes: Prevent and Fight Breast Cancer with Smart Nutrition and Powerful Foods

By Joe Correa CSN

www.ingramcontent.com/pod-product-compliance
Lightning Source LLC
Chambersburg PA
CBHW030256030426
42336CB00009B/396